Smoothies for Weight Loss.

80 Delicious Smoothie Recipes

~

The Best Fruit, Veggies, Weight Loss and Diabetes Smoothies

Jenny Morgan

TABLE OF CONTENT

Introduction

I want to thank you and congratulate you for purchasing this recipe book.

Smoothies are a tasty, delectable and delicious part of our daily dietary choices. Whether taken as a healthy alternative to the proliferation of calorie-empty drinks, meal replacements, or as part of programmed weight loss regimens, this flexible blend of organic antioxidant-rich ingredients is here to stay. Seeing how smoothies have evolved from the simple fruit-and-ice slush of its early days to the sophisticated blends and flavors of today, we realize that while there are many recipes to choose from, there is much room for flexibility and personal creativity in whipping up this particular culinary masterpiece. As you trek through the world of smoothies, you will see the recipes as guides, since it can be easily adjusted to cater to individual tastes, age and even medical conditions. So read on and get caught up in the magical world of smoothies.

History of Smoothies

Smoothies are a product of the 20th century. The concept is thought to have originated from Latin America, mainly Brazil which grows soft, pulpy and fleshy tropical fruits in abundance. Then known as "fruit slush," its early version was made primarily of a combination of shaved fruit, fruit juice and ice.

It was not until 1930 that Steve Poplawski invented what was to be later known as the *blender*. In the late 30's, Fred Waring marketed Poplawski's invention of what was to be popularized as the *Waring blender*. Waring also made some alterations on the blender, increased the speed of its functions including the speed of cutting blades. Then, he sold his invention to various businesses which sold milkshakes. For example: bars, soda foundations, drugstores etc. In the mid-60's, the craze caught on among the California beachgoers and the blended thick frozen drinks made from citrus juices, strawberries and ice evolved into the early version of today's smoothie.

Other cultures also enjoy smoothies in different forms: Indian *lassi* uses a mango-strawberry blend with yoghourt and ice; Mediterranean and Middle Eastern versions known as *sharbat* prefer a yoghourt-honey blend combined with a range of fresh fruits.

In recent developments, the Vita Mix, a powerful blender able to grind nuts and raw vegetables to a smooth paste was introduced. It came out in the market and revolutionized the world of smoothie making.

The Benefits and Advantages of Smoothies

Fruits and vegetables are part of the foundation of our life. They contain molecules that dictate our cells at the DNA level how to respond to various stimuli. If we are taking wholesome green, yellow, or purple smoothies, made of wholesome fresh ingredients, our cells also respond accordingly. They become energetic and healthy. Smoothies offer many benefits and advantages:

- *NO AGE LIMIT.* Smoothies can be enjoyed by people of all ages. Babies over 6 months of age can enjoy banana smoothies combined with milk formula, either by itself or combined with their favorite cereal. The elderly, who are often plagued by mastication and digestive problems, can enjoy their favorite smoothie any time of the day. Anyone in-between can incorporate a regular or occasional smoothie as a quick energy booster.

- *EASE OF PREPARATION.* Smoothies are the easiest to prepare. Armed with a blender, some cut up juicy fruit, fresh or frozen, ice, shaved or crushed, fruit juice and sweetener of your choice (unsweetened is an option), plus a quick buzz and you are ready to go.

- TIME-SAVER. Smoothies can be prepared in the shortest time. Imagine being in a rush early in the morning and having to prepare breakfast for hubby, kids and yourself. Grabbing your blender and ingredients, adding oats and cereals of choice and you have your nutritious meal in just a few minutes. This beats cooking anytime, and also works at dinner and snack time. No more pots and pans and plates to wash; less utensils too!

- *ALLOWS ADVANCE PREPARATION.* Smoothie ingredients can be prepared and measured in advance in cubes, plops or in small containers, and frozen until ready to use.

- *MINIMAL MAINTENANCE.* The blender is the main equipment needed in smoothie preparation, which needs very simple maintenance. Remove the jar, rubber ring, blades and cover parts; wash in sudsy water and rinse well with a teaspoon of vinegar or squeeze of lemon to remove all traces of soap and keep the glass parts sparkling clear.

- *PROVIDES A HEALTHY SOLUTION TO HEALTH ISSUES.* Flexibility of smoothies allows adjustments to be made for health issues such as diabetes and cancer, and to supplement the needs of pregnant women. The hospital dietary osterized feeding (OF) is a smoothie which incorporates fruit, cereals, and vegetables with milk, juice or clear broth.

A Great Meal Replacement

Smoothies may be considered as a great meal replacement for people on the go. It offers the option of increased fiber as well as a flexible choice of fruits and vegetables, incorporated with a bit of cereal, a measure of protein powder, blended with fruit juice, fresh milk or yoghourt and sweetened with Stevia, Agave, honey or other sweetener of choice. It may be enjoyed by students and professionals alike, and anyone too busy to squeeze in a meal between schedules, or want a light, easily absorbable alternative to a regular meal.

Substituting a smoothie for a regular meal is acceptable once in a while, like say, breakfast or as a quick snack while on the go. Some smoothie advocates, however, advise an almost total meal replacement which would result in stringent calorie restriction, resulting in adverse effects which we want to avoid altogether.

With the right shake at meal time, you can get the benefits of a complete meal, and even lower your metabolic rate by as much as 25%, save calories from fatty food, balance your blood sugar level and let the body go into fat burning mode, and increase your energy level – all these without being plagued by hunger pangs and the familiar energy slump and hungry feeling just an hour after you have eaten.

NOTE: You are your body's best judge – eat sensibly, get sufficient sleep, exercise, and treat yourself to a smoothie to replace any meal of the day.

A Perfect Method to Lose Weight

Each individual is unique and with personalized requirements because each person's body has different needs. As a weight watcher's tool, there are some ingredients that you will need to limit or avoid in your smoothies.

- Canned fruit or vegetables went through processing, often with added calories and lower nutritional value. Opt for do-it-yourself fresh or frozen with a low calorie index

- Dairy products like milk, ice cream and yoghourt are full of calories. Opt for plain full fat Greek yoghourt and raw milk.

- Fruit juice are low in nutritional value and high in added calories

- Protein powders are often used for bulk and weight gain. Stick to natural nuts, seeds, Greek yoghourt and agar or unflavored gelatin.

- Sweeteners like honey and maple syrup should be used in moderation; avoid sugar totally. Stevia and agave are natural sweeteners.

For weight-watchers, smoothies are a perfect way to have a meal without sacrificing nutrition, but going on a full smoothie diet is not recommended. Imbalances can occur, and while you will lose weight, it is a temporary or quick fix which will not last. Low calorie index fruit, low fat yoghourt, or whey protein powder combined with healthy fat such as avocado or coconut oil, and green vegetables spiced up with nuts, seeds, cilantro, ginger or any spice of your choice; produce a green smoothie, which is the weight-watcher's choice.

From past times, people learned the value of greens and that green herbs were good for food. Green smoothies will help not only to keep our weight down; it will also keep us healthy and preserve youth. This is attributed to the high plant collagen content which builds up the skin, so that there will be less sagging even with weight loss.

Green smoothies are chock full of easily absorbable vitamins and minerals which extend benefits on a cellular level, and curb hunger pangs without ingesting empty calories. They are also full of amino acids which are building blocks of body's cell regeneration and repair. You may use any green vegetable without strong smell, such as cucumbers, zucchini, carrots or green bell peppers. This is, actually, in line with the suggestion from the health sector to eat one third of our food raw to be able to access those vitamins and minerals which are lost through water, cooking and even ordinary exposure to heat.

Added fiber makes one feel fuller faster and the best thing about it is that you control the ingredients. For example, when starting a diet, you need to test the proportions of protein to see how your body responds to it, and make adjustments based on your findings. The body responds differently to the different classes of vegetables; cruciferous vegetables, for instance, produces flatulence in some people.

A word of warning: the use of green smoothies for weight loss is not supported by the Food and Drug Administration. It is best not to use the same greens too many times in a row, since some greens are toxic in high doses; also some greens are gas formers which may encourage flatulence in some people.

An Important Source of Energy

Our body needs energy to function properly, meet its physical demands and help deal with stressors. Unlike the popular energy drinks in the market today that quickly beef up your energy with a high caffeine level then put you in a slump a few minutes later, smoothies do the exact opposite.

To top it all, not only do they perk up your energy level like a time release capsule without the old familiar slump that leaves you feeling washed-out, they leave you feeling refreshed. With every sip come the benefits that accrue on a large scale by feeding your body on a cellular level; smoothies are easily digestible, its nutrients absorbable and simple. It is a great way to power up your life without compromising your health.

Dr. Ann Wigmore, who invented green smoothies, advocates different types of smoothies – bitter ones like kale and spinach, which are blood cleansers aside from being energy boosters; sweet tender greens such as lettuce and sprouts are enjoyed by many; and some swear by the inclusion of mustard greens which prevent clogging of arteries because of its sulforaphane content. There is no hard and fast rule, so it is still dependent on personal choice.

Smoothies are Full of Antioxidants

Because smoothies are mainly fresh fruit and vegetables, they are bursting with disease-preventing antioxidants. When cell equilibrium is disrupted because of the wrong kind of diet and exposure to free radicals, it opens the door to the entry of different kinds of illnesses such as:

- Cardiovascular disease,

- Diabetes,

- Cancer,

- Alzheimer's disease,

- Inflammatory diseases and others which may benefit from antioxidants' mechanism of action, such as aging.

These are prevented by enzyme and phytonutrient-rich *antioxidants* which prevent autoxidation and inhibit the formation of free radicals which cause cell death. There are synthetic antioxidants such as butylated hydroxytoluene and butylated hydroxyanisole, Phenolic antioxidants, fat-soluble vitamin E, water-soluble vitamin C and plant extracts which are effective in the appropriate matrix, dosage and environment. However, it has been found that excessive antioxidant levels may have the opposite effect and inhibit recovery and adaptation mechanisms.

Antioxidant-rich smoothies have a high *Anthocyanins* (from Greek: (anthos) = flower + (kyanos) = blue) content which are plant chemicals that are found to be 40 times more potent than Vitamins A and C! If you take 40 doses of synthetic Vitamin C and A, toxicity would occur. But it isn't so with antioxidant fruits, which would act as elimination agents of these toxins. The only deterrent to ad libitum enjoyment of fruits would be their sugar content, which would have a negative effect on hyperglycemia, but you can make informed choices by opting for ingredients with low glycemic index.

Fruit Recipes

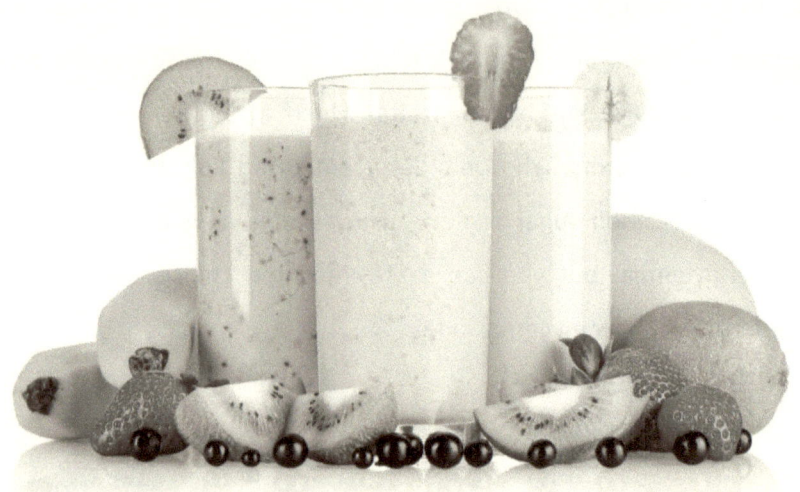

Kiwi and Pineapple Smoothie

Tropical and freeing smoothie, if you like blending fruit flavors; you will love this one.

Serves: 2
Prep time: 5 min

Ingredients:
- Half cup of frozen vanilla yogurt
- 6 strawberries
- 1 kiwi
- 1 banana
- ¾ cup of pineapple and orange juice

Directions:
1. Place the ingredients in a food processor and blend them on high speed until they become smooth and thick.
2. Allow it to chill in the fridge for some time then serve it and enjoy.

Peaches and Strawberries Smoothie

This smoothie is made of simple fresh fruits which makes it delicious and healthy at the same time.

Serves: 4
Prep time: 10 min

Ingredients:
- 2 Peaches
- 1 cup of mango and orange juice
- 2 cups of ice
- 1 quart of strawberries
- 1 chopped banana

Directions:
1. In a blender, combine the banana with strawberries and peaches then blend them well.
2. Add the mango and orange juice with ice cubes to the mix and blend them well
3. Serve it immediately and enjoy.

Berries and Peaches Smoothie

This smoothie is so refreshing and if you are not peach fan, you can always replace it with pear.

Serves: 2
Prep time: 10 min

Ingredients:
- 16 ounces of sliced peaches
- 10 ounces of frozen and mixed berries
- 2 tablespoons of honey

Directions:
1. Blend all the ingredients together on high speed until you are satisfied.
2. Garnish it with some dry fruits and enjoy.

Orange and Mango Smoothie

Delicious flavor and cheerful as well as bright color that gives this smoothie a seat among the best smoothies ever!!!!!

Serves: 1
Prep time: 10 min

Ingredients:
- 1 mango cut into chunks
- 1 chopped banana
- 1 cup of non-fat vanilla yogurt
- 1 cup of orange juice
- 4 ice cubes

Directions:
1. Blend the mango with banana and vanilla yogurt, orange and ice cubes until they become smooth and thick on high speed.
2. Drink it with a straw and enjoy

Mocha and Vanilla Smoothie

This is a cool cold mocha smoothie that is surprisingly so tasty!!!!!!!!!!

Serves: 1
Prep time: 10 min

Ingredients:
- 3 tablespoons of instant coffee with mocha flavor
- 3 tablespoons of granulated sugar
- 1 cup of crushed ice
- ¾ cup of milk
- 1 teaspoon of vanilla extract

Directions:
1. Blend the milk, ice and coffee with vanilla and sugar on high speed until it becomes creamy and smooth.
2. Garnish it with some cacao powder on top and enjoy.

Orange and Vanilla Smoothie

This smoothie is so easy and quick to make, not to mention that it is also full of vitamin C. You can drink daily and you will never get tired of it.

Serves: 4
Prep time: 10 min

Ingredients:
- 3 large oranges cut into chunks
- 6 cups of orange juice
- 3 cups of vanilla yogurt
- Half teaspoon of cinnamon powder
- 8 ice cubes

Directions:
1. Blend everything on high speed until they become creamy and smooth.
2. Serve it immediately and enjoy.

Lemon and Strawberry smoothie

So refreshing and cool, it is perfect for a sunny and hot day to quench your thirst.

Serves: 2
Prep time: 10 min

Ingredients:
- 8 ounces of lemon yogurt
- 10 large strawberries
- 1/3 cup of orange juice
- 4 ice cubes

Directions:
1. Freeze 7 strawberries in a plastic bag or container for 1 h then set aside.
2. In a blender, blend all the ingredients until they become thick.
3. Cut the 3 left strawberries into small cubes or chunks then add them to the smoothie and serve it immediately.

Mango and Peach Smoothie

This one is one of the tastiest and healthiest smoothies that you can come across, as it can also aids in weight loss by keeping feeling full for a long period of time.

Serves: 2
Prep time: 10 min

Ingredients:
- 1 sliced mango
- 1 sliced peach
- Half cup of orange juice
- Half cup of vanilla soy milk
- 4 ice cubes

Directions:
1. In a food processor or a blender, process the mango with peach, orange, milk and ice cubes until they become smooth and creamy like a purée.

Vanilla and Mango Smoothie

This is a smoothie that will also keep you filled and refreshed. It's creamy and smooth and tastes great.

Serves: 2
Prep time: 10 min

Ingredients:
- 1 cup and half of chopped mango
- ¼ cup of vanilla yogurt
- ¾ cup of chilled milk
- 4 ice cubes
- ¼ teaspoon of vanilla extract

Directions:
1. Blend all the ingredients well on high speed until you are satisfied with it.
2. Serve it right away and enjoy.

Pear and Banana Smoothie

The combination of pears and cinnamon is beyond what words can describe, it is so delightful and dreamy.

Serves: 2
Prep time: 10 min

Ingredients:
- 2 pears cut into 4 pieces
- 1 chopped banana
- Half cup of vanilla yogurt
- 1 cup of milk
- 1/8 teaspoon of nutmeg
- Half teaspoon of cinnamon
- 4 ice cubes

Directions:
1. In a food processor, combine the ice cubes with yogurt, pears chunks, cinnamon, nutmeg and milk then blend them for at least 1 min until they become smooth.
2. Once the time is up, add the banana to them and blend them until they become creamy and thick.
3. Serve it with some pear chunks and enjoy.

Chocolate and Cherries Smoothie

Easy and elegant, if you were in a hurry this smoothie will make your day.

Serves: 2
Prep time: 10 min

Ingredients:
- 3 frozen and chopped bananas
- 2 cups of chocolate soy milk
- 2 cups of dark sweet and frozen cherries

Directions:
1. Process all the ingredients in a blender until it become smooth like a purée.
2. Garnish it with some berries on top and enjoy it.

Cantaloupe and Raspberries

When you find some good deals in the cantaloupe season, don't hesitate to benefit from it because you will need it once you taste this unbelievable smoothie.

Serves: 2
Prep time: 10 min

Ingredients:
- 1 cup of raspberries
- Half cup of skinless and diced cantaloupe
- Half cup of plain yogurt
- 3 tablespoons of sugar
- 4 ice cubes

Directions:
1. Dup the cantaloupe with sugar, yogurt, ice cubes and banana in a blender and blend them until they become creamy and smooth.
2. Serve it immediately and enjoy.

Mint and Pineapple Smoothie

This frosty smoothie is full of bright and beautiful colors in addition it tastes amazing.

Serves: 2
Prep time: 10 min

Ingredients:
- 3 frozen strawberries
- 1 cup of frozen diced pineapple
- 3 fresh chopped mint leaves
- ¼ cup of skinless and seedless grapes
- ¼ cup of unsweetened apple sauce
- 1 tablespoon of lime juice

Directions:
1. In a blender, combine the lime juice with grapes and apple sauce and blend them well for at least 1 min.
2. Once the time is up, add the rest of the ingredients and pulse them a few times until the strawberries and pineapple because like small chunks.
3. Allow it to chill in the fridge for some time then serve it and enjoy.

Mixed Berries Smoothie

One gulp is all what stops this smoothie from being your favorite, so go ahead and try it.

Serves: 2
Prep time: 1h 10 min

Ingredients:
- 1 banana
- Half cup of mixed and frozen berries
- 1 cup of almond milk
- Half cup of fresh cranberries

Directions:
1. Blend all the ingredients in a blender until they become smooth then allow them to chill in the fridge for almost 1 h.
2. Once the time is up, serve your smoothie and enjoy.

Flax Seed and Banana Smoothie

This smoothie is packed with omega 3 and fibers, which makes it and perfect and healthy smoothie for everyone.

Serves: 2
Prep time: 10 min

Ingredients:
- 1 cup of frozen strawberries
- 1 cup of low fat vanilla soy milk
- Half cup of frozen and chopped banana
- 1 tablespoon of flax seed meal

Directions:
1. Place all the ingredients in a blender and blend it well until it becomes like a purée.
2. Allow it to chill in the fridge for some time then serve it and enjoy.

Kiwi and Tangelos Smoothie

Sometime you stumble among a good deal of kiwi and you end up with lot of it, the smoothie is a great use of it and you will be craving it each day.

Serves: 4
Prep time: 10 min

Ingredients:
- 5 peeled and chopped kiwis
- 1 cup and half of plain yogurt
- 1 and ¼ cup of soy milk
- 1 cup of fresh mix of berries
- 2 tangelos
- 1 banana
- 1 tablespoon of sugar
- 1 sprig of mint leaves
- 6 ice cubes

Directions:
1. In a food processor, blend the kiwi with banana, tangelos and soy milk, kiwis and yogurt, berries, ice cubes and mint until they become thick and smooth.
2. Add the sugar gradually until you are satisfied with its sweetness.
3. Serve it right away or keep it in the fridge and enjoy.

Apple and Peanut Butter Smoothie

This is a unique and very refreshing smoothie that is perfect for summer.

Serves: 3
Prep time: 10 min

Ingredients:
- 1 cup of low fat vanilla yogurt
- 1 cup of apple juice
- 1 cup of chunky apple sauce
- 2 tablespoons of smooth peanut butter
- ¼ cup of caramel ice cream
- 1 tablespoon of caramel ice cream topping

Directions:
1. In a plastic container, poor the apple juice and allow it to freeze for 2 h then break it into pieces and set it aside.
2. In a blender, combine the apple sauce with yogurt ¼ cup of caramel ice cream and peanut butter and blend them until they become creamy and smooth.
3. Poor the smoothies into 3 glasses and garnish it with the left tablespoon of caramel ice cream topping.

Papaya and Vanilla Smoothie

This smoothie is so creamy, delicate and delicious; it'll be one of your favorites for sure.

Serves: 2
Prep time: 10 min

Ingredients:
- 2 cups of peeled and diced papaya
- 1 cup of vanilla yogurt
- 2 cups of ice
- 2 cups of milk
- 2 tablespoons of cream cheese
- ¼ cup of sugar
- ¼ cup of sweet condensed milk

Directions:
1. Place all the ingredients in a blender and blend them until you are satisfied with it.
2. Serve it immediately and enjoy it.

Mango and Pineapple Smoothie

This smoothie is delicious, not to mention that is bright yellow color will enlighten your mood and give you a good start to your day.

Serves: 2
Prep time: 10 min

Ingredients:
- Half cup of fresh chopped mango
- Half cup of diced fresh pineapple
- Half cup of coconut water
- Half cup of orange juice
- 1 banana
- 1 chopped sprig of chocolate mint
- 1 teaspoon of fresh lime juice
- 4 ice cubes

Directions:
1. Dump all the ingredients in a food processor and blend them until they become smooth and creamy on high speed.
2. Serve it immediately and enjoy.

Acai and Cacao Smoothie

This smoothie is so healthy because it contains some powerful antioxidants, not to mention that it is gluten free and low on carbs.

Serves: 2
Prep time: 10 min

Ingredients:
- 2 cups of fresh berries
- 24 ounces of acai juice
- Half cup of pasteurized egg white
- 3 tablespoons of cacao powder
- 2 tablespoons of cinnamon
- ¼ cup of truvia natural sweetener
- 1 cup of apple cider

Directions:
1. In a food processor or a blender, blend all the ingredients together until they become thick and creamy.
2. Allow it to chill in the fridge for some time until you are satisfied and enjoy.

Crunchy Tea and Pineapple Smoothie

Everybody knows that tea is good for you and how many benefits it provides to our bodies, so this a great chance to consume it in a different way.

Serves: 2
Prep time: 10 min

Ingredients:
- 1 peeled and chopped kiwi
- 1 cup of chopped pineapple
- 1 cup of boiling water
- 1 bag of 2 g of green tea
- 1 large and peeled orange
- 3 tablespoons of non-fat Greek yogurt

Directions:
1. In a bowl, place the boiling water with a tea bag and allow it to stay for 5 min.
2. Once the time is up, remove the tea bag and allow it to chill in the fridge for at least 1 h.
3. When the time is over, dump all the ingredients in a blender until you are satisfied with it.
4. Serve it cold and enjoy.

Banana and Flax Seed Smoothie

If you are looking for a smoothie that will be good in any diet, here is one. It is full of calcium, protein and fiber as well.

Serves: 2
Prep time: 10 min

Ingredients:
- Half cup of frozen strawberries
- Half cup of non-fat plain yogurt
- Half cup of frozen and chopped banana
- Half cup of non-fat milk
- 2 tablespoons of protein powder
- 1 tablespoon and half of flax seed
- 1 teaspoon of honey

Directions:
1. Blend all the ingredients together in a blender until you have a thick, creamy and smooth.
2. Serve it with strawberries or berries on top and enjoy.

Weight Loss Smoothie Recipes

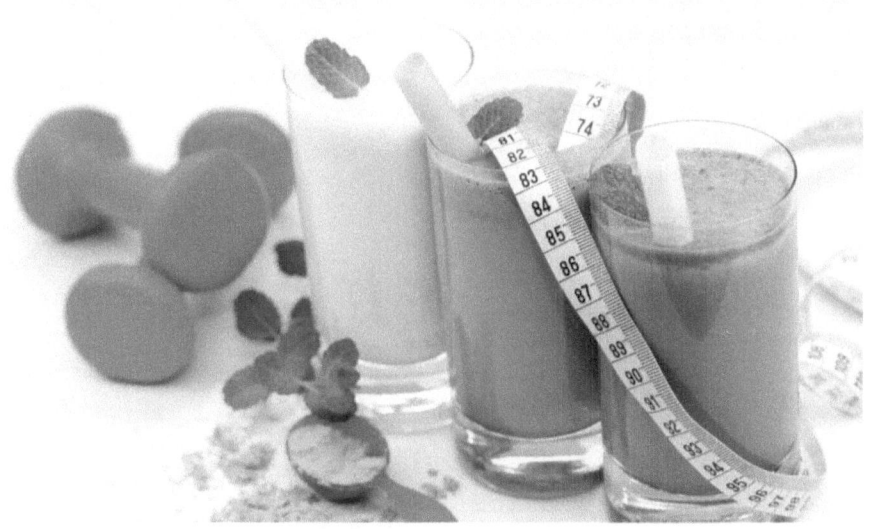

Chocolate and Banana Smoothie

With this recipe, you will be able to eat chocolate and stay healthy at the same time; so don't waste the chance.

Serves: 2

Prep time: 10 min

Ingredients:

- 1 cup of low fat smooth peanut butter
- 1 cup of non-fat milk
- 12 ice cubes
- 2 tablespoons of chocolate whey protein powder
- 1 banana

Directions:

1. In a food processor, combine all the ingredients together and blend them well.
2. Serve it right away or keep it in the fridge and enjoy.

Vanilla and Espresso Smoothie

Vanilla and espresso? You will probably think that this is a horrible combination; Try it and you probably chance your mind.

Serves: 2

Prep time: 10 min

Ingredients:

- 1 cup of frozen vanilla yogurt
- 4 teaspoons of cacao powder
- 2 shot of espresso
- 8 ice cubes

Directions:

1. Dump all the ingredients in a blender and mix them well until it becomes smooth.
2. Serve it cold and enjoy.

Lemon and Watermelon Smoothie

I love water lemon; it is one of my favorite fruits ever. I couldn't wait to share with you this mouthwatering recipe.

Serves: 2

Prep time: 10 min

Ingredients:

- 6 cups of chopped and seedless watermelon
- 1 cup of lemon sherbet
- 12 ice cubes

Directions:

1. In a blender, blend well half of the ingredient and set them aside.
2. Repeat the process then serve it cold and enjoy.

Blueberries and Banana Smoothie

If you are vegan, this smoothie is perfect for you as it is full of protein that your body needs.

Serves: 2

Prep time: 10 min

Ingredients:

- 1 cup of chopped banana
- Half cup of soy Protein
- 8 ounces of water
- Half cup of frozen Blueberries
- 1 tablespoon of honey
- 1 tablespoon of flaxseeds oil

Directions:
1. Blend all the ingredient in a blender until they become smooth then allow them to chill in the fridge for 15 to 30 min or more.
2. Serve it cold with some grated dark chocolate on top and enjoy.

Blueberries and Vanilla Smoothie

This smoothie is like a slap on the face to wake you up, and make you open your eyes and see how you can drink amazing smoothies and at the same time maintain a perfect and healthy body.

Serves: 2

Prep time: 10 min

Ingredients:

- 1 cup of soy milk
- 1 cup of frozen blueberries
- 1 cup of fresh blueberries
- 6 ounces of vanilla yogurt
- 1 tablespoon of flaxseed oil

Directions:

1. In a blender, blend the soy milk with yogurt, fresh and frozen blueberries for at least 1 min.
2. Once the time is up, add the flaxseed oil to the mix and blend them for another 30 second.
3. Serve it and enjoy.

Avocado and Mango Smoothie

The combination of these ingredients will stimulate your taste buds and keep them asking for more.

Serves: 2

Prep time: 10 min

Ingredients:

- ¼ cup of vanilla yogurt
- 1/5 cup of mango juice
- ¼ cup of diced fresh mango
- ¼ cup of mashed avocado
- 6 ice cubes
- 1 tablespoon of lime juice
- 1 tablespoon of sugar or honey

Directions:

1. Blend all the ingredients well in a blender until they become smooth.
2. Serve it cold and enjoy.

Spinach and Pear Smoothie

Spinach and Pear? Really?
That's what everyone say once they hear about this combination, but they taste it...I'll let you answer that question yourself.

Serves: 2

Prep time: 10 min

Ingredients:

- 2 cups of spinach leaves
- 15 green grapes
- 6 ounces of non-fat Greek yogurt
- 1 chopped pear
- 2 tablespoons of lime juice
- 2 tablespoons of chopped avocado

Directions:
1. Place all the ingredients in a blender and blend them until they become smooth and creamy.
2. Allow it chill in the fridge for 15 min or more then serve it and enjoy.

Apple and Pecan Smoothie

This smoothie is to die for, try it quickly and let me know what you think.

Serves: 2

Prep time: 10 min

Ingredients:

- 1 chopped apple
- 1 cup of unsweetened coconut milk
- ¼ cup of unsalted pecans
- 1 tablespoon of coconut butter
- 1 tablespoon of coconut protein powder
- ¼ teaspoon of cinnamon
- 2 teaspoons of honey
- ¼ teaspoon of nutmeg
- 4 ice cubes

Directions:

1. Blend all the ingredients together until they become smooth then serve your smoothie right away and enjoy.

Green Tea and Blueberries Smoothie

Both green tea and blueberries have a magnificent ability to burn fat and provide your body with all the necessary vitamins.

Serves: 2

Prep time: 10 min

Ingredients:

- 2 cups of blueberries
- 12 ounces of fat free yogurt
- 2 green tea bags
- 12 of fat free yogurt
- 3 ice cubes
- 3 tablespoons of almonds
- 3 tablespoons of ground flax seeds

Directions:

1. Place the tea bags in 3/4 cup of water and allow it to cool down.
2. Process all the ingredients in a food processor then serve it and enjoy.

Chocolate and Chitosan Smoothie

Two in one, in this smoothie you will be able to satisfy yourself with dark chocolate that will unexpectedly help you burn fat.

Serves: 2

Prep time: 10 min

Ingredients:

- 1000 mg of Chitosan
- 1 cup of water
- Half banana
- Half cup of frozen blueberries
- 1 teaspoon of unsweetened cacao
- Half pack of milled flaxseed
- 1 tablespoon of whey protein
- 5 ice cubes

Directions:
1. Dump all the ingredients in a food processor and mix them until you're satisfied.
2. Serve it right away and enjoy.

Vanilla and Cherry Smoothie

Dr. Oz offers this smoothie as one of the best to help you lose fat.

Serves: 1

Prep time: 10 min

Ingredients:

- 5 ice cubes
- Half cup of soy milk
- Half banana
- 1 cup of cherry juice
- Half cup of soy milk
- ¼ teaspoon of vanilla extract

Directions:

1. Place all the ingredients in a food processor and blend them well.
2. Serve it cold and enjoy.

Pineapple and Coconut Smoothie

With this smoothie, you will feel like you are on a tropical island and lose weight at the same time.

Serves: 2

Prep time: 10 min

Ingredients:

- 5 ice cubes
- 6 ounces of fat free yogurt
- ¾ cup of diced pineapple
- 1 chopped banana
- 1 cup of spinach
- ¾ of coconut milk
- 2 tablespoons of shredded coconut

Directions:

1. Process all the ingredients until they become smooth then serve cold and enjoy.

Peach and Almond Smoothie

This smoothie is full of fatty acids that helps you burn fat, and it gives you a great burst of energy.

Serves: 2

Prep time: 10 min

Ingredients:

- 2 cups and half of chopped peaches
- 8 ice cubes
- 2 cups of soy milk
- 3 tablespoons of almond butter
- 1 teaspoon of cinnamon
- Tablespoon of sliced almonds

Directions:

1. Place all the ingredients in food processor and blend them until they become creamy and smooth.
2. Garnish it with some sliced peaches then serve it cold and enjoy.

Cucumber and Lime Smoothie

This smoothie is not only heavenly delicious but it also offers you so many benefits and vitamins that your body needs.

Serves: 2

Prep time: 10 min

Ingredients:

- 6 ounces of Greek yogurt
- 3 ice cubes
- 3 mint leaves
- 2 seedless and chopped cucumber
- 2 teaspoons of honey
- Half lime's juice
- 1/8 teaspoon of black pepper

Directions:
1. Put everything in a food processor until you are satisfied with it.
2. Garnish it with some chopped mint leaves and enjoy.

Melon and Kale Smoothie

For a quick and easy method to burn fat, melon, spinach and kale are great choices.

Serves: 2

Prep time: 10 min

Ingredients:

- 14 cubes of melon
- 1 frozen banana
- 1 cup of baby kale
- 1 cup of baby spinach leaves
- Half cup of milk
- Half cup of non-fat Greek yogurt
- 5 ice cubes

Directions:
1. Place all the ingredients in a food processor and blend them well.
2. Serve it with some small chunks of melon and enjoy.

Strawberries and Oat Smoothie

4 words: you will love it. This smoothie is one of the best.

Serves: 2

Prep time: 10 min

Ingredients:

- 1 cup of chopped strawberry
- 1 cup of milk
- 1 cup of ice
- Half cup of yogurt
- Half cup of oats
- Half cup of ground flax seed meal

Directions:

1. This is a wonderful and perfect breakfast that contains all the vitamins your body needs to function well.

Parsley and Cucumber Smoothie

This smoothie is the perfect way to start your day, as it contains loads of vitamins that will keep you full and satisfied most of the day.

Serves: 2

Prep time: 10 min

Ingredients:

- 2 cups of spinach
- Half bunch of chopped parsley
- 1 bunch of mint
- 2 chopped apples
- 3 chopped carrots
- Half chopped cucumber
- ¼ lime
- ¼ pineapple
- ¼ orange
- ¼ lemon

Directions:

1. Dump all the ingredients in a food processor until it becomes smooth.
2. Allow it to chill in the fridge for some time and enjoy.

Tomato and Strawberry Smoothie

There is nothing better than a smoothie that is full of vitamin C to improve and strengthen your immunity.

Serves: 2

Prep time: 10 min

Ingredients:

- 1 skinless tomato
- 2 oranges
- Half cantaloupe
- 1 cup of strawberries
- 5 ice cubes

Directions:

1. Juice the oranges and set them aside.
2. In a blender, process the orange juice with the rest of the ingredients until you are satisfied.
3. Serve it with some sugar powder on top and enjoy.

Berries and Kale Smoothie

This smoothie will not only help you maintain a healthy body, but beautiful and healthy skin as well.

Serves: 2

Prep time: 10 min

Ingredients:

- 1 cup of water
- 5 ice cubes
- ¼ cup of blueberries
- ¼ cup of strawberries
- ¼ cup of raspberries
- ¼ cup of kale

Directions:

1. Blend all the ingredients in a food processor until it becomes creamy or until you are satisfied.
2. Serve it immediately and enjoy.

Vanilla and Berries Smoothie

Perfect taste and amazing benefits is what you get from this smoothie.

Serves: 2

Prep time: 10 min

Ingredients:

- 1 cup of vanilla almond milk unsweetened
- 1 cup of frozen mixed berries
- 1 tablespoon of whey protein powder
- 1 teaspoon of chia seeds
- 1 tablespoon of flaxseed
- Half cup of water

Directions:

1. Dump all the ingredients in a food processor and blend them well.
2. Garnish it with some mix of berries and enjoy.

Orange and Blueberries Smoothie

Drink this smoothie 3 times a day and you will notice that you are losing weight rapidly.

Serves: 1

Prep time: 10 min

Ingredients:

- 35 g of frozen blueberries
- 125 g of frozen raspberries
- 1 scoop of vanilla protein powder
- Half peeled and sliced orange
- 1 tablespoon of ground linseeds
- 4 ice cubes

Directions:

1. In a smoothie maker or a blender, dump all the ingredients and blend them well until they become smooth and thick.
2. Serve it right away and enjoy.

Veggies Smoothie Recipes

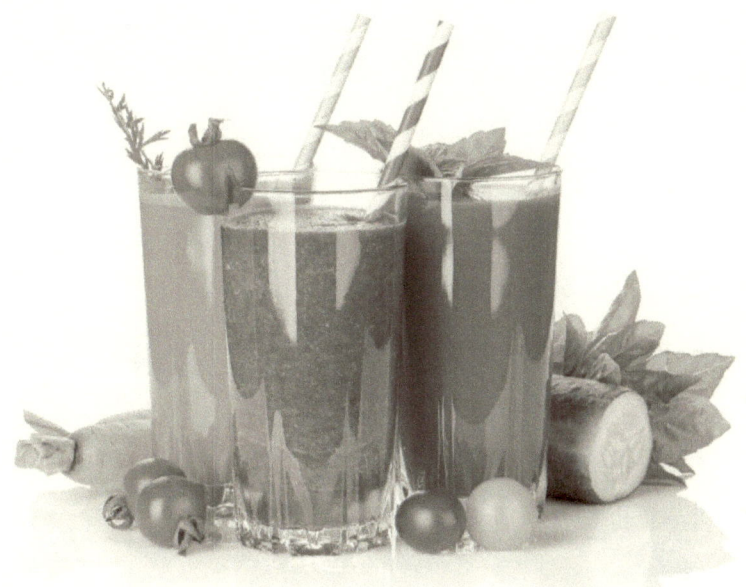

Pumpkin Smoothie

Pumpkin lovers. Try this recipe right now and see for yourself how amazing it is.

Serves: 2

Prep time: 10 min

Ingredients:

- 16 ounces of pumpkin purée
- 2 cups of milk
- ¼ cup of sugar
- 2 teaspoons of cinnamon
- 4 ice cubes

Directions:

1. Blend the ingredients in a blender until you are satisfied.
2. Serve it immediately and enjoy.

Zucchini and Cacao Powder

To be honest, this recipe might look bizarre but it is insanely tasty, but only courageous people will dare to try it.

Serves: 2

Prep time: 10 min

Ingredients:

- 1 cup of frozen and grated zucchini
- Half cup of sugar
- 1 cup of half and half
- ¼ cup of chopped peanuts
- 2 frozen bananas
- 2 tablespoons of cacao powder
- 4 ice cubes

Directions:

1. Blend all the ingredients in a food processor until they become thick and smooth.
2. Garnish it with some cacao powder and serve it immediately.

Sweet Potato Smoothie

Amazing and adjustable smoothie that will still taste wonderful with any addition you choose.

Serves: 1

Prep time: 9 h10 min

Ingredients:

- 1 sweet potato
- 1 banana
- 2 cups of soy milk
- ¼ teaspoon of cinnamon
- 4 ice cubes

Directions:

1. Bake the potato for 1 h in the oven on 350 f then peel it and allow it to cool down.
2. Place the potato in the fridge for an overnight then dump all the ingredients in a food processor and blend them well until they become smooth and creamy.
3. Serve it cold and enjoy.

Pineapple and Kale Smoothie

Youngsters and adults both will love this smoothie, it is a pure bliss.

Serves: 2

Prep time: 10 min

Ingredients:

- 1 cup and half of frozen pineapple chunks
- 1 chopped banana
- 1 cup of chopped kale
- 1 cup of almond milk
- 4 ice cubes

Directions:

1. In a blender, mix all the ingredients together and serve them cold then enjoy.

Carrot and Kiwi Smoothie

So exotic and tropical, it is the best smoothie for a hot day.

Serves: 2

Prep time: 10 min

Ingredients:

- 1 chopped kiwi
- 1 cup of chopped carrots
- 1 cup of ice cubes
- 1 cup of chopped pineapple
- 1 chopped banana

Directions:

1. Place the ingredients in your blender and process them for 1 min until it becomes creamy and thick.
2. Serve it right away and enjoy.

Broccoli and Grapes Smoothie

Broccoli and grapes are magical and are two great combinations that you definitely should try.

Serves: 2

Prep time: 10 min

Ingredients:

- 1 cup of seedless grapes
- 2 cups of chopped broccoli
- Half cup of water
- 1 small chopped cucumber
- The juice of one lime
- 4 ice cubes

Directions:

1. Combine all the ingredients in a blender and process them until you are satisfied.
2. Serve it cold and enjoy.

Mint and Cacao Smoothie

The best of the best, nothing can conquer the combination of the cacao and mint flavor.

Serves: 2

Prep time: 10 min

Ingredients:

- 10 chopped fresh mint leaves
- 1 cup chopped of spinach leaves
- 1 frozen and chopped banana
- Half cup of cold coconut milk
- ¼ cup of cacao seeds
- 1 gram of stevia powder
- 1 teaspoon of peppermint extract
- Half cup of water
- 3 ice cubes

Directions:

1. Blend all the ingredients except for the banana in a blender for 30 seconds.
2. Once the time is up, keep blending them and add to them one by one the pieces of banana.
3. Serve it cold and enjoy.

Beet and Carrots Smoothie

This vegetable smoothie is full of many important vitamins, not to mention that is a great source of energy for your body.

Serves: 2

Prep time: 10 min

Ingredients:

- 1 cup of water
- 1 cup of spinach leaves
- Half skinless beet
- Half skinless orange
- Half skinless lime
- 1/3 cup of chopped baby carrots
- 1/3 cup of cauliflower florets
- 1/3 cup of broccoli florets
- 1 stalk of celery
- ¼ cup of blueberries
- 1 tablespoon of chia seeds
- 1 tablespoon of honey
- 3 ice cubes

Directions:

1. On high speed, blend all the ingredients together for 1 min until it becomes thick and smooth.

2. Serve it cold and enjoy.

Peach and Cabbage Smoothie

Hurry and make your own smoothie, because this recipe is to die for.

Serves: 4

Prep time: 10 min

Ingredients:

- 1 chopped carrot
- 1 cup of sinless grapes
- 1 cup of sliced and frozen peaches
- ¾ cup of chopped cabbage
- ¼ cup of water
- 4 ice cubes

Directions:

1. Process all the ingredients in a blender until you are satisfied.
2. Serve it cold and enjoy.

Jalapeno and Spinach Smoothie

If you are a jalapeno fan then you will absolutely like this smoothie, as it combine the best of the sweet and hot flavor.

Serves: 2

Prep time: 10 min

Ingredients:

- 2 chopped bananas
- 1 cup of frozen chopped mango
- 2 cups of baby spinach leaves
- Half teaspoon of chopped jalapeno

Directions:

1. Blend the ingredient on high speed for 1 min until they become thick and creamy.
2. Serve it immediately and enjoy.

Carrot and Ginger Smoothie

Everybody knows how much ginger and carrots benefit our bodies. These ingredients are known to strengthen your immunity system.

Serves: 2

Prep time: 10 min

Ingredients:

- 4 chopped baby carrots
- ¼ cup of water
- ¼ cup of chopped almonds
- ¼ cup of Spirulina
- 1 chopped beet
- 4 ice cubes
- 1 chopped inch of ginger

Directions:

1. In a blender, process the beet with ginger, carrots and water for 1 min.
2. Once the time is up, add the rest of the ingredients and blend them until they become thick and smooth.
3. Serve it cold and enjoy.

Tomato and Basil Smoothie

This recipe might look like a salad but it is actually delicious and healthy.

Serves: 2

Prep time: 10 min

Ingredients:

- 2 large basil leaves
- 1 cup of spinach leaves
- Half chopped tomato
- Half cup of chopped frozen mango
- Half cup of ice cubes

Directions:

1. Blend all the ingredients together until they become smooth and thick.
2. Serve it cold and enjoy.

Cabbage and Apple Smoothie

Mouthwatering combination of healthy ingredients, what more could you ask for?

Serves: 2

Prep time: 10 min

Ingredients:

- 1 cup of chopped cabbage
- 1 cup of seedless red grapes
- 1 cup of chopped apple
- 1 chopped carrot
- 4 ice cubes
- Half cup of water
- Tablespoon of fresh chopped ginger

Directions:

1. Place all the ingredients in a food processor and process them until they become smooth and creamy.
2. Serve it with some grapes and enjoy.

Healthy Salad Smoothie

You can always get rid of the jalapeno if you don't like spicy food, but you should try this recipe because of its many health benefits.

Serves: 2

Prep time: 10 min

Ingredients:

- 1 chopped tomato
- 1 bell pepper
- 1 jalapeno
- 3 handfuls of spinach
- 2 cups of water
- 1 clove of garlic
- 2 stalks of celery
- ¼ onion
- ¼ cucumber
- 2 teaspoon of Spirulina
- 1 teaspoon of kelp
- 4 ice cubes

Directions:

1. In a food processor, dump all the ingredients and blend them until they become smooth and thick. You can always add some water to it if you are not okay with it.

Celery and Kale Smoothie

This is a very healthy recipes, it is known for its multitude of vitamins. Great benefits to your immunity system and also for healthier skin.

Serves: 1

Prep time: 10 min

Ingredients:

- 2 kale leaves
- 1 skinless lemon
- 1 skinless and chopped apple
- 1 small chopped cucumber
- 2 chopped celery stalks
- 1 handful of spinach
- 3 ice cubes
- 2 teaspoons of honey
- 1 cup of cold water

Directions:

1. Using a juicer, juice the apple, kale, spinach, cucumber, kale and lemon.
2. Dump all the ingredients in a blender and blend them until they become creamy and smooth.
3. Garnish it with some grapes then serve it and enjoy.

Turmeric and Coconut Smoothie

I never heard of a smoothie with turmeric, so why not to try it. This combination might seem odd but it super healthy and mouthwatering.

Serves: 1

Prep time: 10 min

Ingredients:

- 1 banana
- 2 egg yolks
- Half teaspoon of turmeric
- 1 teaspoon of grated fresh ginger
- 1 tablespoon of coconut oil
- 2 teaspoons of lemon juice
- 1/3 cup of coconut milk
- 1 tablespoon of honey
- 3 ice cubes

Directions:

1. In a food processor, blend all the ingredients except for the egg yolk on high speed for 1 min.
2. In a small bowl, beat the egg yolk then add it to the blender.
3. Serve it right away or place in the fridge and enjoy.

Caramel and Pumpkin Smoothie

The mix of caramel and pumpkin is absolutely delightful and irresistible.

Serves: 1

Prep time: 10 min

Ingredients:

- 1 cup of vanilla ice cream
- 2 crushed vanilla wafers
- Half cup of pumpkin purée
- ¾ cup of milk
- ¾ teaspoon of pumpkin spice
- 3 teaspoons of ice cream caramel topping
- 3 ice cubes

Directions:

1. In a blender, blend the ice cream with milk and spice until they become smooth.
2. Dip the serving glass in the ice cream caramel then dip it again in the crushed wafers and set it aside.
3. Serve the smoothie with some pie spice on top and enjoy.

Lemon and Parsley Smoothie

This smoothie is quite amazing as it cleans the liver and the gallbladder in addition to many other benefits.

Serves: 1

Prep time: 10 min

Ingredients:

- 3 kale leaves
- 3 stalks of celery
- 1 inch peeled ginger
- 1 large beet
- 2 green apples
- 2 lemons
- 1 cucumber
- 1 bunch of dandelion greens
- 1 bunch of parsley

Directions:

1. Place all the ingredients in a blender and process them until they become smooth.
2. Allow the smoothie to chill in the fridge for 15 min or more then serve it cold and enjoy.

Broccoli and Cottage Cheese Smoothie

Cottage cheese, pineapple and broccoli are an awesome combination, it is simply divine.

Serves: 2

Prep time: 10 min

Ingredients:

- 1 cup of apple juice
- 2 cups of ice
- Half cup of broccoli florets
- Half cup of fresh pineapple
- Half cup of wheatgrass
- 3 tablespoons of cottage cheese
- 1 teaspoon of fresh grated ginger

Directions:

1. In a blender, blend all the ingredients and enjoy.

Cucumber and Avocado Smoothie

Cucumber and avocado are a very close veggies, once they are combined they become mind blowing.

Serves: 1

Prep time: 10 min

Ingredients:

- Half avocado
- Half sliced cucumber
- 2 bunches of baby spinach
- 8 ice cubes
- 4 skinless limes
- Half teaspoon of cinnamon
- 1 tablespoon of liquid stevia
- Half cup of water

Directions:

1. In a blender, blend all the ingredients in a food processor on high speed for 1 min.
2. Once the time is up, serve it and enjoy.

Spinach and Strawberry Smoothie

So yummy, and the important thing is that your kids will love it.

Serves: 1

Prep time: 10 min

Ingredients:

- 2 cups of chopped spinach
- Half cup of ice
- 2 cups of frozen strawberries
- 1 chopped banana
- 2 tablespoons of honey

Directions:

1. Blend all the ingredients on high speed for almost 1 min.
2. Once the time is up, garnish the smoothie with some fruit chunks and enjoy.

Jenny Morgan

Diabetes Smoothie Recipes

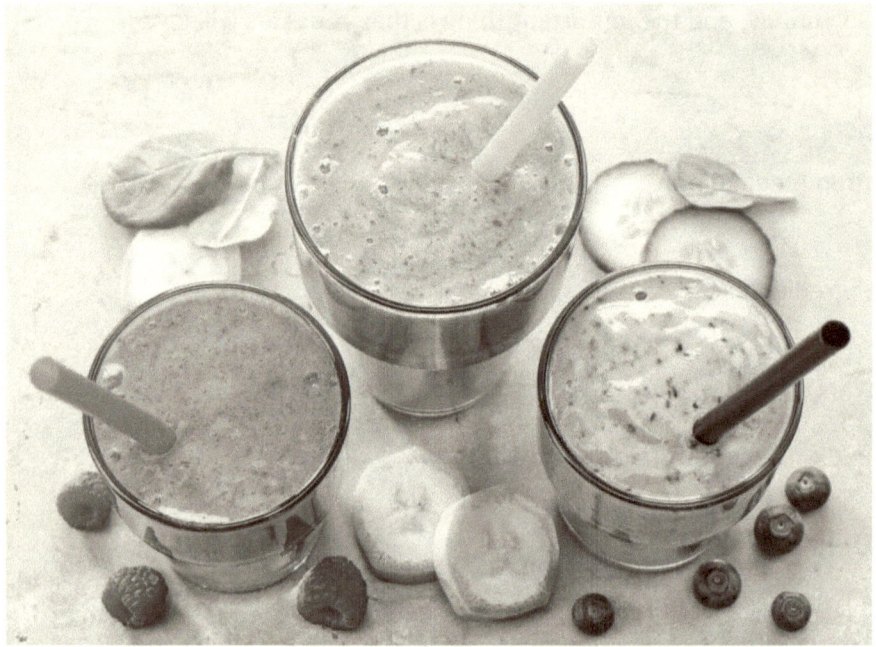

Almond and Blueberries Smoothie

People with diabetes must be very careful when they choose their foods, but that doesn't mean that they must give up on eating this delicious smoothie.

Serves: 1

Prep time: 10 min

Ingredients:

- 3 droppers of liquid stevia
- 1 cup of non-fat plain Greek yogurt
- Half cup of almond milk
- 1 cup and half of frozen blueberries
- ¾ cup of completely pasteurized egg whites
- 3 ice cubes

Directions:

1. Place all the ingredients in a blender and blend them until you get a thick and smooth smoothie.
2. Serve it immediately and enjoy.

Mango and Pineapple Smoothie

The banana and mango in this smoothie add all the sweetness that you need without having to add sugar or a sweetener, and the best thing about it is that it is fat free.

Serves: 1

Prep time: 10 min

Ingredients:

- Half peeled and chopped mango
- Half chopped banana
- Half cup of citrus fat free and sugar free yogurt
- 4 ice cubes
- 2/3 cup of skimmed milk
- 2 teaspoons of protein powder

Directions:

1. Blend everything in a blender or smoothie maker until it becomes thick and creamy.
2. Serve it immediately and enjoy.

Almond and Honey Smoothie

This smoothie is a super and perfect breakfast because it is full of proteins and fibers that will load your body with energy and help you get through the day.

Serves: 1

Prep time: 10 min

Ingredients:

- 2 tablespoons of honey
- 2 tablespoons of wheat germ
- 1 cup and half of blueberries
- 1 cup of ice cubes
- Half cup of fat free plain yogurt
- ¼ cup of chopped and slivered almonds
- 2 tablespoons of unsweetened almond milk

Directions:
1. Blend all the ingredient together until you are satisfied with it.
2. Serve your smoothie immediately and enjoy.

Peaches and Almond Milk Smoothie

This is perfect smoothie if you are having a long day and you need something to boost you energy and replace your regular coffee.

Serves: 2

Prep time: 10 min

Ingredients:

- 1 cup of mixed frozen peaches and strawberries
- 1 cup of almond milk
- 3.5 ounces of Greek yogurt

Directions:

1. Blend all the ingredients at once until they become smooth and creamy then serve it right away and enjoy.

Strawberries and Spinach Smoothie

WOW!!!! When you try this marvelous smoothie that is what you will say because it is simply awesome.

Serves: 2

Prep time: 10 min

Ingredients:

- Half cup of strawberries
- Half cup of blueberries
- 2 cups of spinach
- 1 tablespoon of chocolate protein powder
- 1 tablespoon of ground flax seed
- One bunch of either raw walnuts or pumpkin seeds
- 2 tablespoons of dry chia seeds
- 1 teaspoon of cinnamon
- 4 crushed ice cubes

Directions:

1. In a small bowl or cup, soak the chia seeds until they become like gelatin.
2. In a blender, blend all the ingredients until they become smooth and thick then serve it immediately and enjoy.

Chocolate and Peanut Butter Smoothie

So rich on fiber and protein but at this same time this smoothie will raise all your expectations and introduce you to a whole new level of deliciousness.

Serves: 1

Prep time: 10 min

Ingredients:

- 8 ounces of crushed ice cubes
- 1 small sliced banana
- Half cup of fat free sour cream
- 3 tablespoons of low fat peanut butter
- 2 teaspoons of unsweetened cacao powder
- 4 teaspoons of Splenda sugar substitute

Directions:

1. In a blender, food processor or smoothie make blend all these ingredients for at least 30 sec or more until you are satisfied.
2. Once the time is up, poor your smoothies in glasses and garnish it with banana chunks then serve it and enjoy.

Cacao and Date Smoothie

This natural and kind of raw smoothie is awesome because it tastes like chocolate and is naturally sweetened.

Serves: 1

Prep time: 10 min

Ingredients:

- 3 ice cubes
- 1 date
- 5 almonds
- 1 cup of almond milk
- 1 frozen and chopped banana
- 1 tablespoon of raw cacao

Directions:
1. Dump all the ingredients in a food processor until it becomes smooth and rise up to your liking.
2. Garnish it with some raw cacao then serve it and enjoy.

Avocado and Kale Smoothie

Almost everybody know how much green smoothies or fruits and veggies generally are important for our bodies, so this is a perfect opportunity to consume delicious and healthy smoothie.

Serves: 2

Prep time: 10 min

Ingredients:

- 16 ounces of chilled water
- 2 cups of kale
- 2 cups of frozen mix of peaches, mango and pine apple or any other fruits
- 1 cucumber
- 1 stalk of celery
- 1 frozen and chopped banana
- Half avocado
- 1 peeled lemon

Directions:

1. Process everything in a smoothie make or food processor for 1 min.
2. When the time is up, garnish it with some berries and enjoy.

Ginger and Chia Seeds Smoothie

This smoothie is full of vitamins and benefits that are perfect for healing and preventing diabetes, and at the same time they so delicious.

Serves: 2

Prep time: 10 min

Ingredients:

- 1 tablespoon of chia seeds
- 1 tablespoon of coconut oil
- 1 tablespoon of raw cacao powder
- 1 tablespoon of dry goji berries
- 1 the juice of 1 ginger root
- 8 ounces of water or more
- 2 teaspoon of ground cinnamon
- 1/8 teaspoon of cayenne pepper
- ¼ teaspoon of turmeric
- Half cup of fresh sprouts
- 3 frozen cherries
- ¼ cup of frozen blueberries
- 2 frozen pieces of banana

Directions:

1. In a blender, blend the coconut oil with ginger juice, water and cayenne pepper, turmeric, cacao powder and cinnamon for at least 30 sec
2. At the same time, soften the goji berries and chia seeds for later use.
3. Once the time is up, add the frozen and goji berries with sprouts and cherries, banana and chia seeds to the blender and started on low moving higher.
4. Blend the ingredients for 1 min and add to them some chilled water in case it became too thick for your liking.
5. Serve it immediately with some berries on top and enjoy.

Oats and Almond Smoothie

If you are having a high blood sugar, this smoothie will help your problem and keep you healthy.

Serves: 2

Prep time: 10 min

Ingredients:

- 6 ounces of unsweetened almond milk
- 2 frozen strawberries
- 3 tablespoons of organic rolled oats
- 1 tablespoons of flax seed
- 1 tablespoons of raw cacao
- 1 bunch of spinach
- 3 sliced of cucumber
- Half stalk of celery
- 1 teaspoon of cinnamon
- 4 ice cubes

Directions:

1. Blend all the ingredients until they become smooth and creamy.
2. Poor the smoothies in glasses then garnish them with some strawberries and enjoy.

Chickweed and Avocado Smoothie

This smoothie will actually help you maintain a healthy level of blood sugar and maintain a healthy body as well.

Serves: 2

Prep time: 10 min

Ingredients:

- Half cup of chilled water
- 1 bunch of chickweed
- 3 spinach leaves
- Half cup of plain yogurt
- Half cup of frozen berries
- Bunch of dandelion greens
- 3 sprigs of mint
- 3 sprigs of parsley
- Half avocado
- 2 teaspoons of soaked chia seeds

Directions:

1. In a food processor, blend all the ingredients well and add to them more water if it is too thick for you or add yogurt to make it thicker.
2. Serve it with some fresh berries on top and enjoy.

Bok Choy and Plum Smoothie

This smoothie is the easiest so far, so give yourself a chance to try it and say good bye to high blood sugar and bad food.

Serves: 1

Prep time: 10 min

Ingredients:

- 1 head of baby bok choy
- 1 pitted red plum
- 1 frozen chopped banana
- ¼ chopped avocado
- 1 cup of chopped kale
- Half cup fat free yogurt

Directions:

1. Just sump all the ingredients in a food processer and blend it on high speed until it becomes creamy and thick.
2. Serve it immediately and enjoy.

Coconut and Lime Smoothie

This tropical smoothie is awesome, not to mention that its amazing vibrant green color is eye catching.

Serves: 2

Prep time: 10 min

Ingredients:

- 1 chopped avocado
- /The juice of 2 limes
- 1 cup of frozen pineapple chunks
- 1 scoop of vanilla protein powder
- 1 cup of coconut water
- 1 teaspoon of fresh grated ginger
- 4 ice cubes

Directions:

1. Dump all the ingredients in your blender and blend them until they become smooth and creamy.
2. Serve it immediately and enjoy.

Aloe Vera and Cherries Smoothie

You will be surprised because this smoothie contain aloe vera, but you will be more surprised to learn that it can prevent diabetes.

Serves: 1

Prep time: 10 min

Ingredients:

- 1 cup of aloe vera gel
- 1 cup of cherries
- 4 ice cubes
- 1 cup of chopped banana
- 1 teaspoon of ground cinnamon

Directions:

1. Process the ingredients until it becomes creamy like a purée for some minutes.
2. Once the time is up, serve it immediately and enjoy.

Banana and Almond Smoothie

Almonds are packed with many vitamins that not only heal you from the inside but from the outside as well. It helps improve the health of your hair and reduces or prevents hair loss. It'll also beautify your skin. Bananas are great anti-aging food. So why don't try this delicious smoothie.

Serves: 1

Prep time: 10 min

Ingredients:

- 1 cup of oranges
- 1 cup of chopped banana
- 4 ice cubes
- Half cup of water
- ¼ cup of almonds
- Half teaspoon of ground cinnamon

Directions:

1. Process all the ingredients until it becomes a creamy and thick smoothie for at least 1 min.
2. When the time is up, serve your smoothie right away and enjoy.

Banana and Tofu Smoothie

The ingredients in this smoothie provide your body with fatty acids, omega 3 and fibers as well, all what you need in one smoothie.

Serves: 1

Prep time: 10 min

Ingredients:

- Half cup of soft tofu
- 1 cup and half of trimmed strawberries
- Half sliced banana
- 2 tablespoons of skim milk
- 2 tablespoons of ground flax seeds
- 1 cup of ice cubes
- 2 teaspoons of honey

Directions:

1. Purée the ingredients in a blender until it become thick and smooth for some min.
2. Once the time is up, serve it with a drizzle of honey on top and enjoy.

Apple and Maple Syrup Smoothie

Combining apple and maple syrup is a magnificent combination that will stimulate your taste buds and show you how some smoothies can be really good.

Serves: 1

Prep time: 10 min

Ingredients:

- 2 cups of baby spinach
- 1 cup of ice cubes
- Half cup of fat free yogurt
- 1 chopped apple
- 1/3 cup of orange juice
- 1 teaspoon and half of maple syrup
- 2 tablespoons of ground flax seed

Directions:

1. In a blender combine the spinach with yogurt and apple, maple syrup, orange juice and flax seed until they become smooth like a purée.
2. Add the ice to the blender and pulse it a few times until it becomes creamy then serve it and enjoy.

Broccoli and Pineapple Smoothie

This smoothie is super awesome; it looks so creamy and smooth. You can use it even as a pudding.

Serves: 1

Prep time: 10 min

Ingredients:

- Half Fuji apple
- Half cup of broccoli florets
- 1 cup of ice cubes
- Half cup of fresh spinach leaves
- Half cup of skim milk
- Half avocado
- Half cup of pineapple chunks
- 2 tablespoons of soaked chia seeds

Directions:

1. Place the ingredients in a smoothie maker or a blender and blend it for 1 min and 30 sec.
2. When the time is up, garnish it with some silvered almond then serve it and enjoy.

Oat Meal and Almond Smoothie

When you drink this smoothie, you will provide your body with 30 per cent of fibers that it needs each day.

Serves: 2

Prep time: 10 min

Ingredients:

- Half cup of ice cubes
- Half cup of free fat plain Greek yogurt
- Half cup of oat meal
- Half cup of frozen blueberries
- Half frozen banana
- ¼ cup of unsalted almonds

Directions:

1. Purée all the ingredients in a blender or smoothie maker until you are satisfied.
2. Serve it right away and enjoy.

Green Grapes and Cabbage Smoothies

This green smoothie contains many antioxidants that not only prevent diabetes but many other diseases as well.

Serves: 1

Prep time: 10 min

Ingredients:

- Half cup of green cabbage
- Half cup of spinach leaves
- Half cup of skim milk
- Chopped carrot
- Half cup of sliced peaches
- Half cup of ice cubes
- Half cup of green grapes
- 1 tablespoon of ground flax seed

Directions:

1. Purée the ingredients in a blender until you are satisfied then serve it immediately and enjoy.

Almond Butter and Raspberries Smoothie

At last but not least, this amazing smoothie will provide your body with all the protein it needs and to help build muscles in the process as well.

Serves: 1

Prep time: 10 min

Ingredients:

- Half cup of frozen raspberries
- 5 unsweetened and frozen strawberries
- Half cup of ice cubes
- 2/3 cup of soy or goat milk
- 1 tablespoon of almond butter
- Half cup of kale
- Half chopped banana
- 1 tablespoon of almond

Directions:

1. Toss the ingredients in a blender and blend them until the smoothie become thick, creamy and smooth.
2. Garnish it with some raspberries then serve it and enjoy.

Conclusion

Thank you again for purchasing this book! I really do hope you found it helpful and love it like I do.

The recipes for these smoothies are like a treasure to me, so I had to share them with you. Words can't describe my love for smoothies. These are not only simple and delicious drinks, they can help you lose weight and improve your overall health as well.

If you like this book or have any comments, your feedback/review is really appreciates.

THANK YOU and ENJOY!